Griefabet

EveryDayGrief Letters
to Wrap Around
your Heart

Karen O. Johnson, MEd.

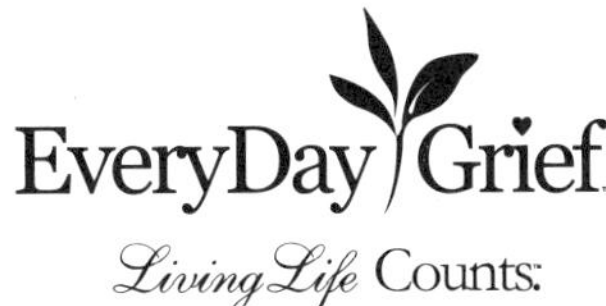

www.Griefabet.com

EveryDayGrief, LLC
PO Box 804
Riverton, Utah 84065
Tel: 801-674-9112
www.griefabet.com

Ordering Information
Quantity sales: Special discounts are available on quantity purchases by corporations, associations, and others. For details, contact EveryDayGrief at the address above.

Individual sales. EveryDayGrief publications are available through www.amazon.com. They can also be ordered from www.griefabet.com or direct from EveryDayGrief at the address above.

Workbook for Helping Professionals
Griefabet Workbook (How to Use Griefabet in Real Counseling Situations) for helping professionals and teachers are available for use. Please contact EveryDayGrief at the address above or visit www.griefabet.com for ordering information.

Orders by U.S. trade bookstores and wholesalers. Please contact EveryDayGrief at the address above.
Printed in the United States of America

Library of Congress Cataloging-in-Publication Data
Johnson, Karen O.
Griefabet: Everyday Grief Letters to Wrap Around your Heart /
Karen O. Johnson, MEd.
p. cm.
Includes bibliographical references
ISBN 978-0-615-39746-7
1. Gift Book. 2. Self-Help. 3. Loss.
4. Mental Health. 5. Grief Counseling. I. Title.

Book design by Ryan Mansfield

Griefabet

is a comfort book for anyone, anytime,
any page, any order, and any day.
It offers support for you and your unique sadness.
Use this book however you desire.
It is like Grief...no rules, no instructions,
no miracle cure, and no role models.
Your Grief is your private rollercoaster and individual
cul-de-sac, and a mighty lonesome state of affairs.
There is no GPS (GriefPathSystem);
you will make your own way with your
personal heartlight and your solitary safari
as you travel inside your heart.

Change is always abrupt
and alters our every breath.
As you patch together a different life,
may you Honor the Past, Embrace the Present,
and Nourish the Future.

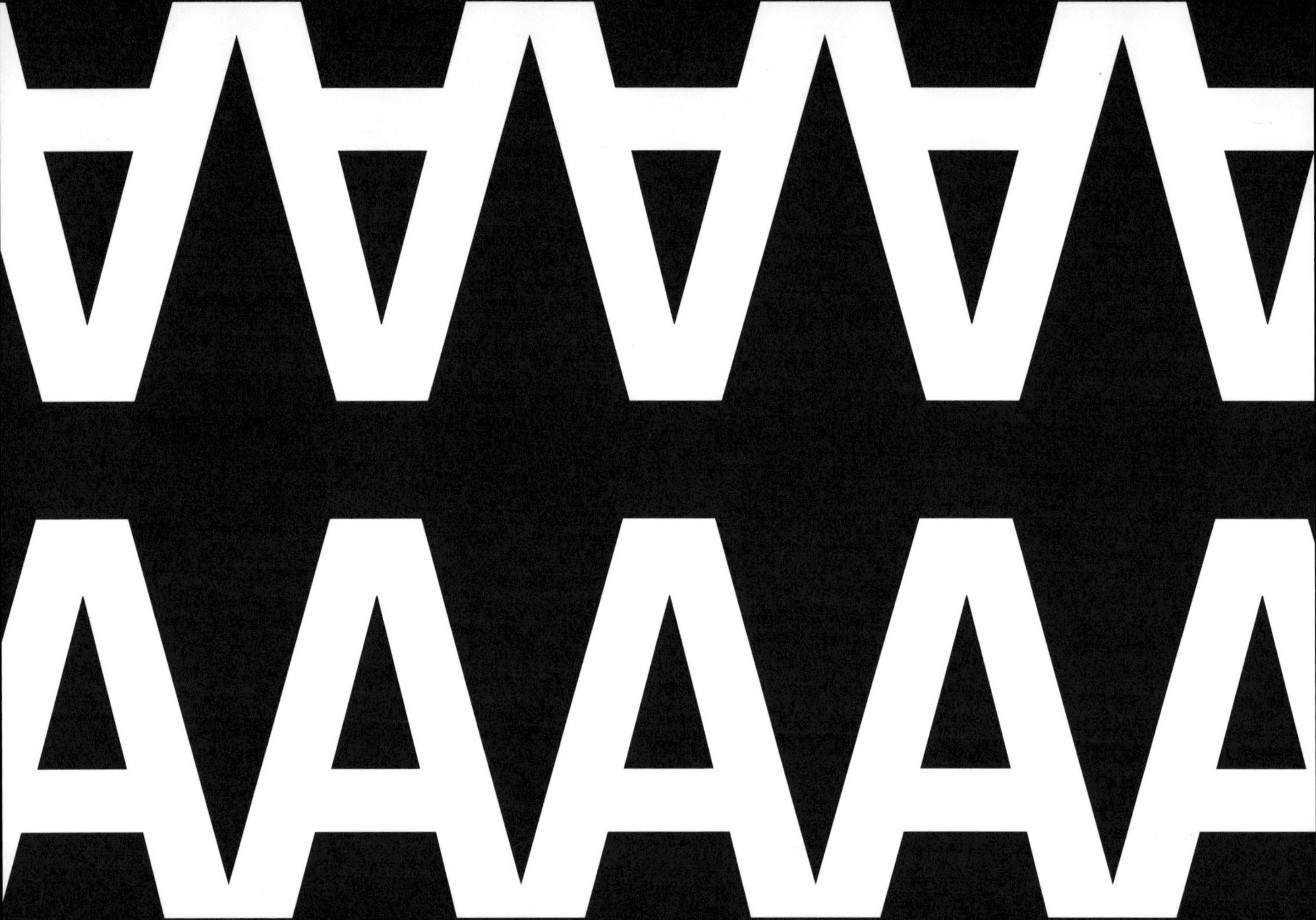

A is for **Anger**

It is okay to feel **A**ngry
that life is not fair.

Attack your garage and throw
marshmallows at it.
Anger unpacked revives **A**djusted dreams.

B is for **Balance**

It is okay to feel **B**ewildered and unsure.

Birdfeeders bring **B**illboards of **B**eauty
in your **B**ackyard.
Balancing yesterday, today and tomorrow
is a **B**eginning.

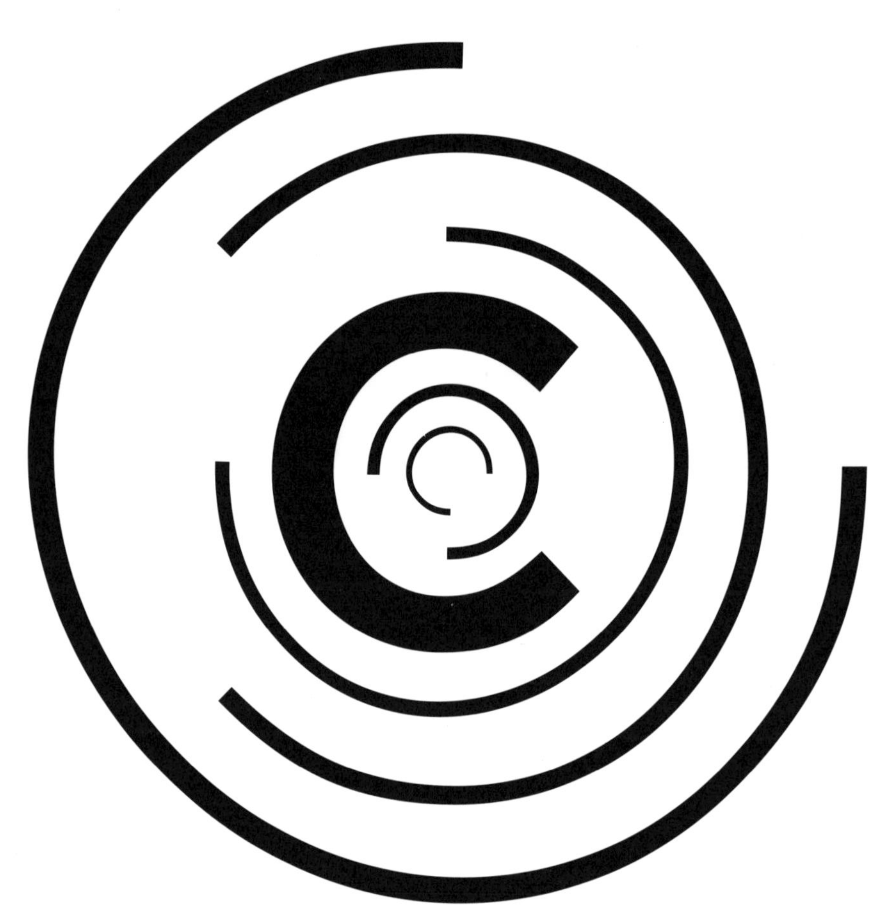

C is for **Craziness**

It is okay to feel **C**razy
amidst so many **C**hanges.

Color using your non-dominant hand.
Create a **C**olorspace to **C**alm the **C**haos.

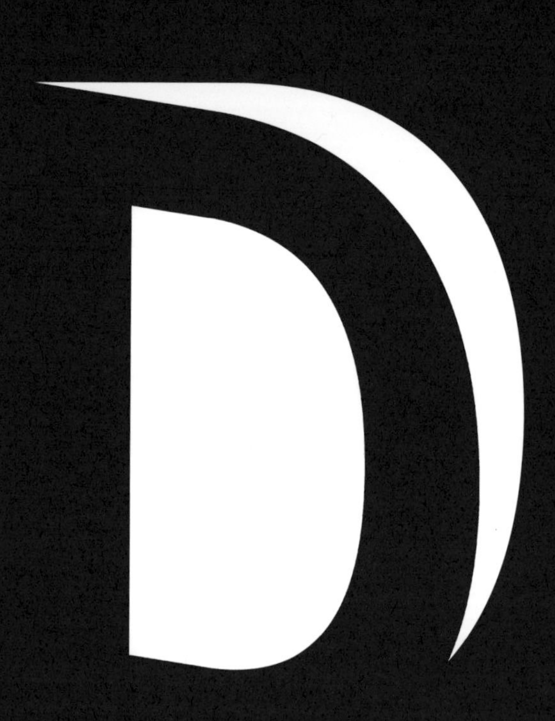

D is for **Discovery**

It is okay to feel **D**ifferent now.

Drive around with no particular **D**estination.
Disappointment is **D**istracting.

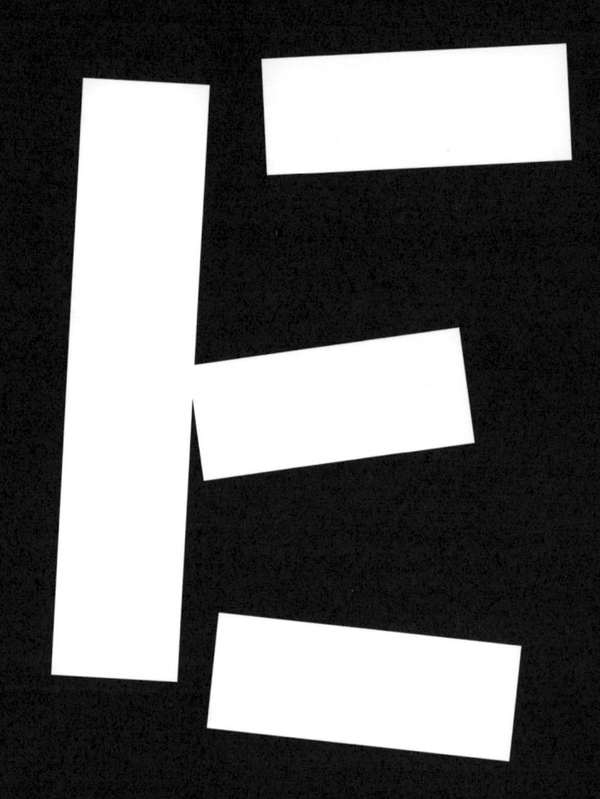

E is for **Empty**

It is okay to wish you could **E**scape broken dreams.

Embrace your pet or stuffed animal.
Endings are **E**xhausting.

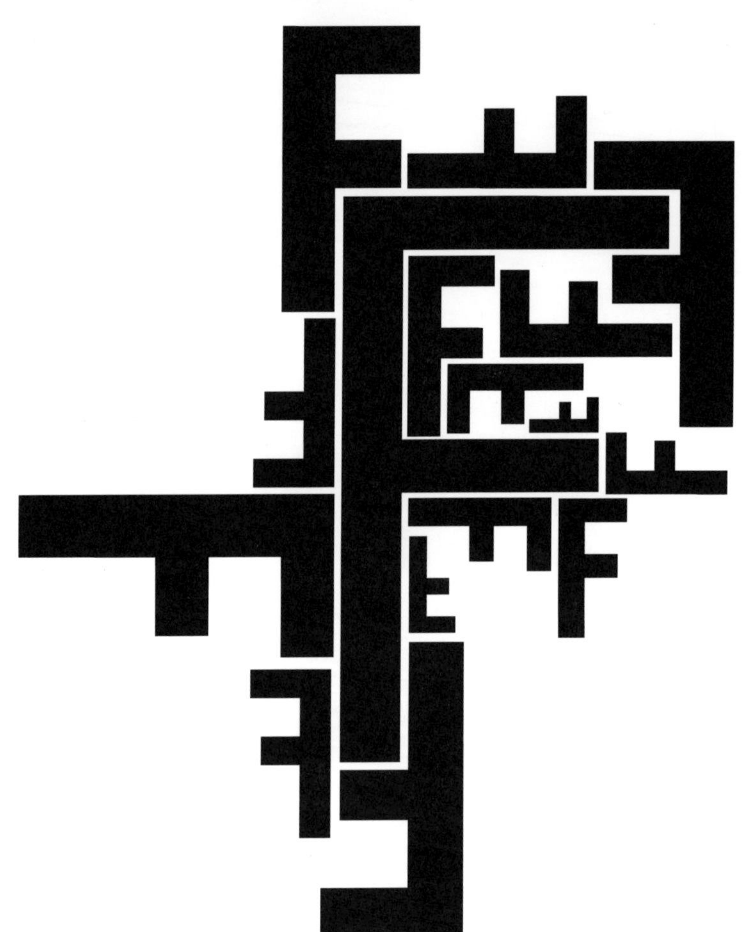

F is for **Feelings**

It is okay to **F**ace what you **F**eel.

Find a Griefspace.
Facing your **F**eelings reduces **F**atigue.

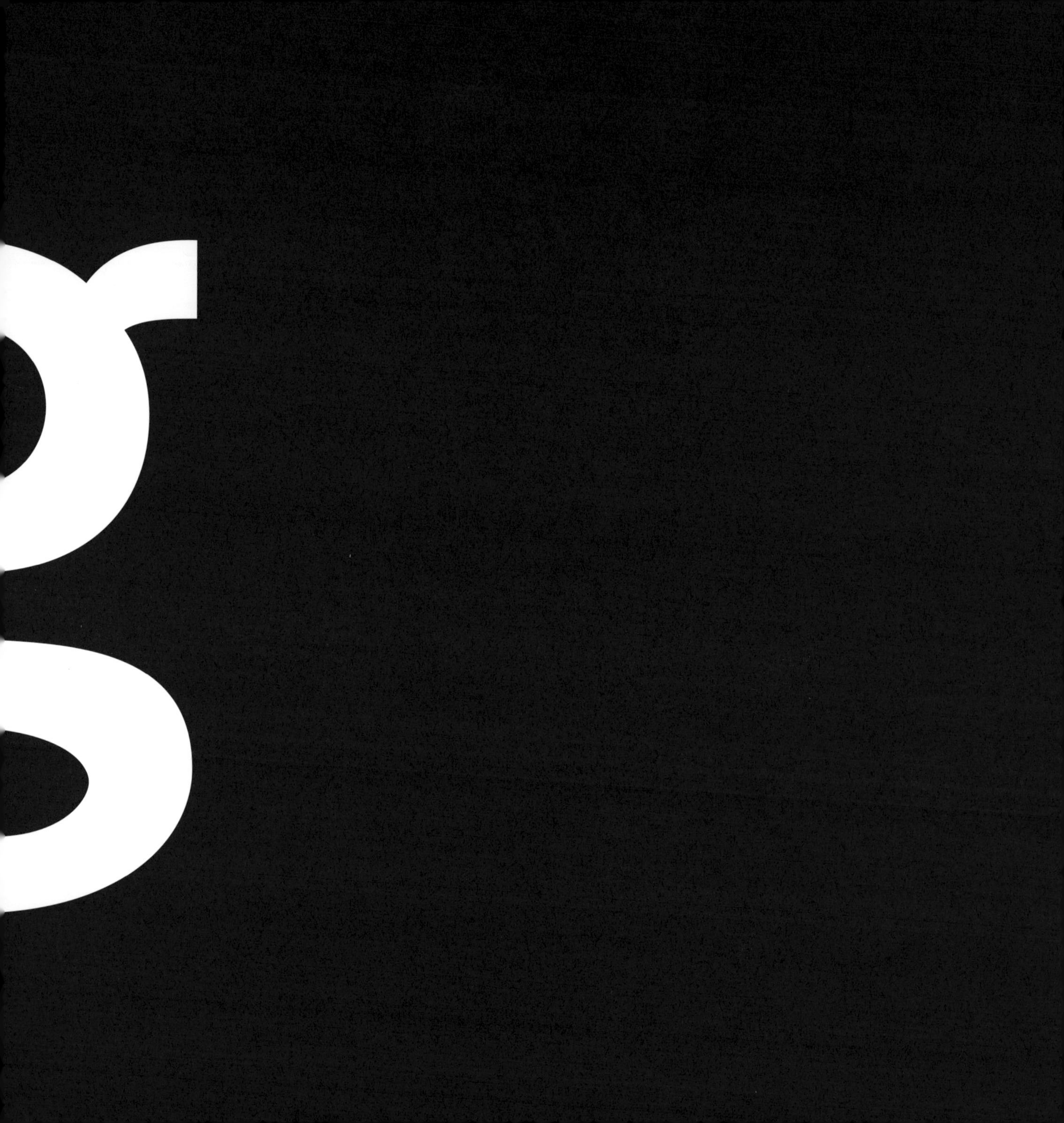

G is for **Good-bye to yesterday**

It is okay to feel **G**ypped.

Grab the **G**rief blanket and wrap it around you.
Getting used to loss is **G**ruesome.

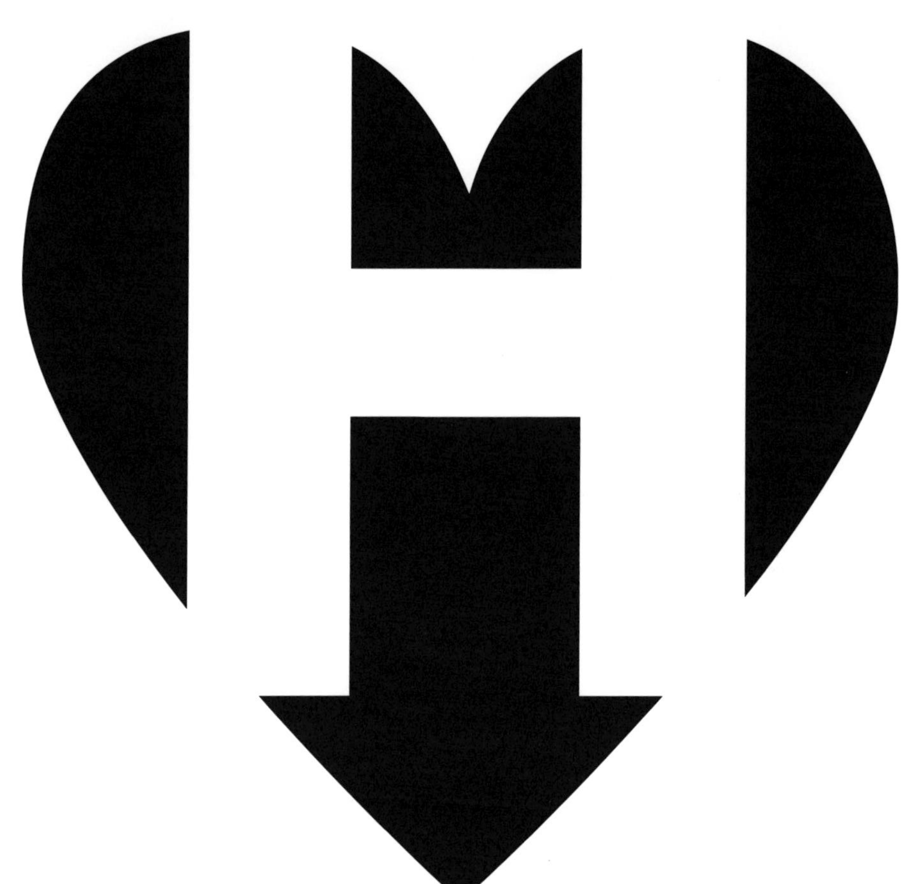

H is for **Hole-in-the-Heart**

It is okay to feel **H**urt and broken-**H**earted.

Hold a piece of paper.
Rip it three times and tape it back together.
Your **H**ead and **H**eart are the same,
yet different now.

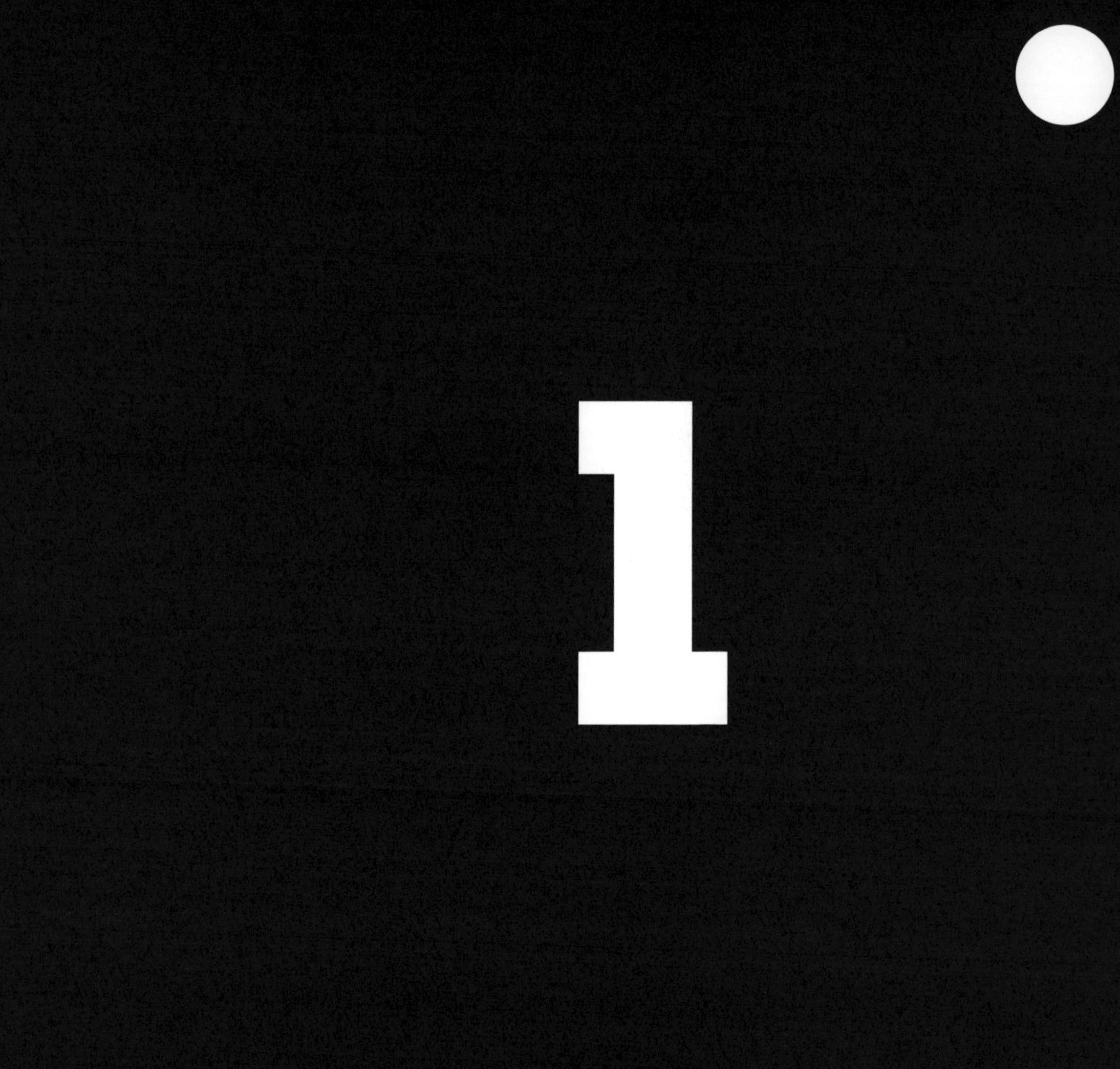

I is for **Identity**

It is okay to feel **I**ncomplete and lost.

Inhale deeply, exhale slowly.
Investigate "Who am **I** now?"

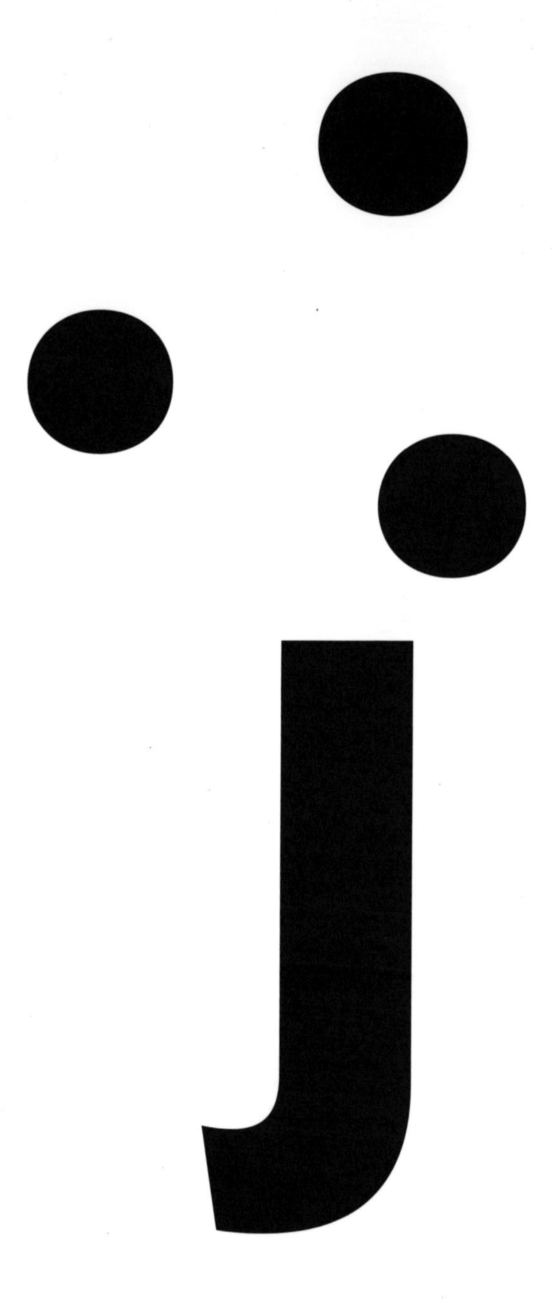

J is for **Juggling**

Journey to people who "really" see you.

Jumpstart your engine and read to a child.
Joy can be re-found and rekindled.

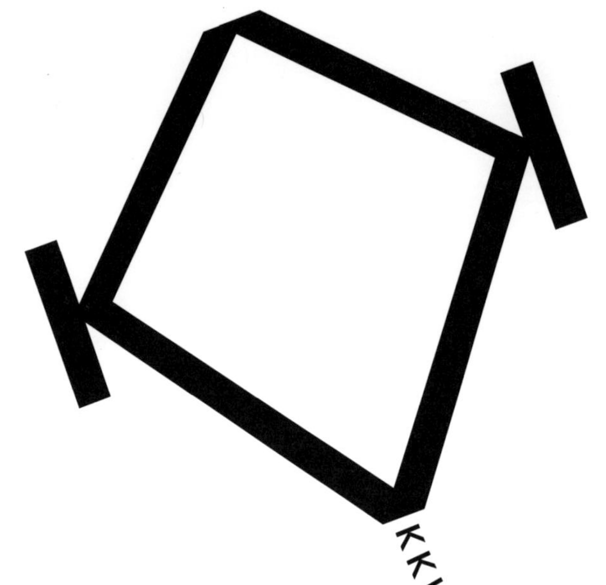

K is for **Kinks**

It is ok to feel motion sick as moods
Kick up and down.

Kite-fly.
Keep your joints moving.

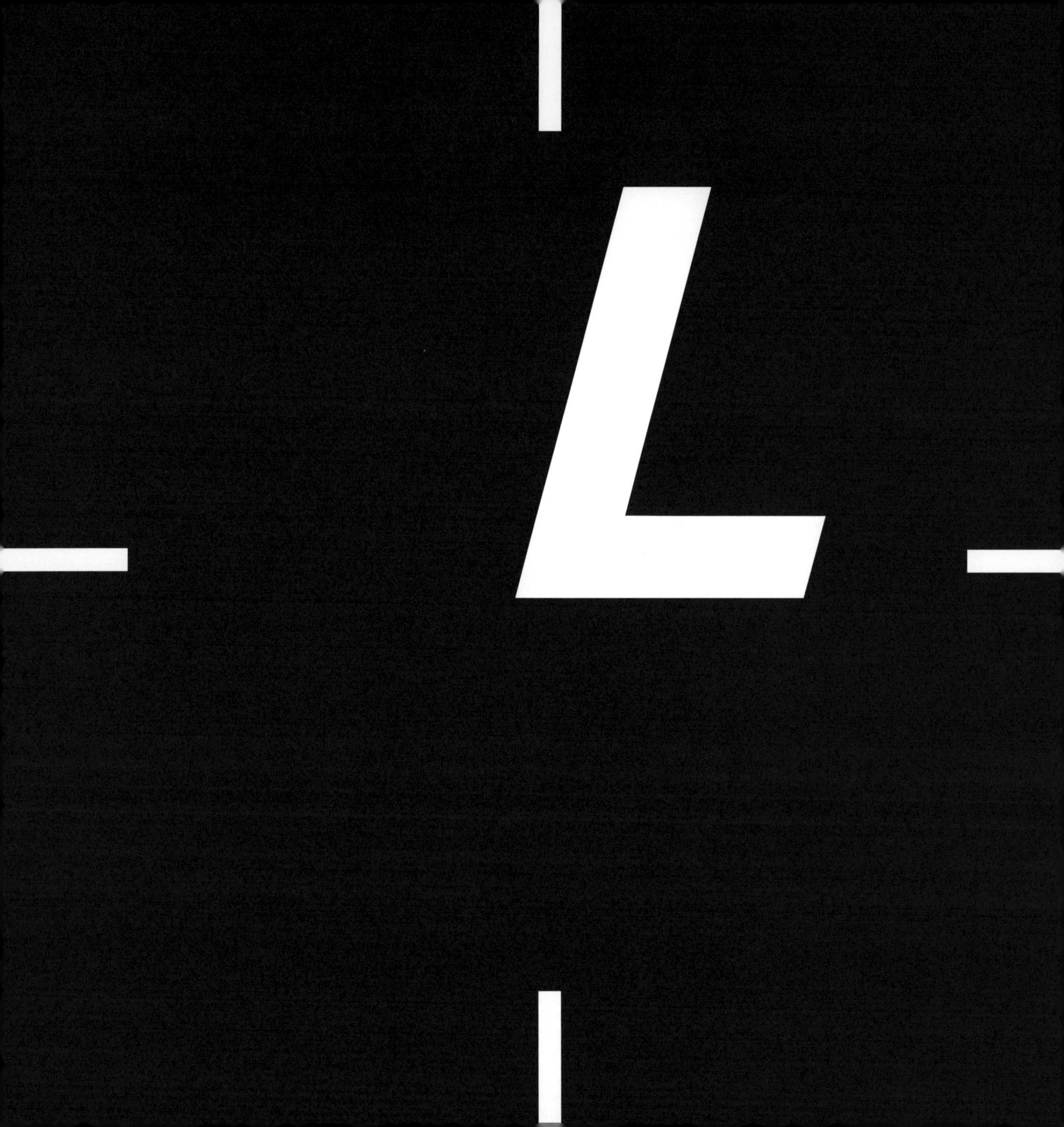

L is for **Leaning in**

It is okay to experience **L**andmines of emotion.

Linger with your grief.
Set a timer and feel the worst you can
until it dings.
Levels of pain **L**essen through hurting.

MMMM

M is for **Memorializing**

It is okay to feel **M**iserable and lonesome.

Magnets on the fridge are a
natural **M**emory board.
Miss them. Their life **M**atters.

N

N is for **Numb**

It is okay to feel paralyzed in GriefLand.

Navigate your imagination
and have a conversation with your loved one.
Newness of life altered is startling.

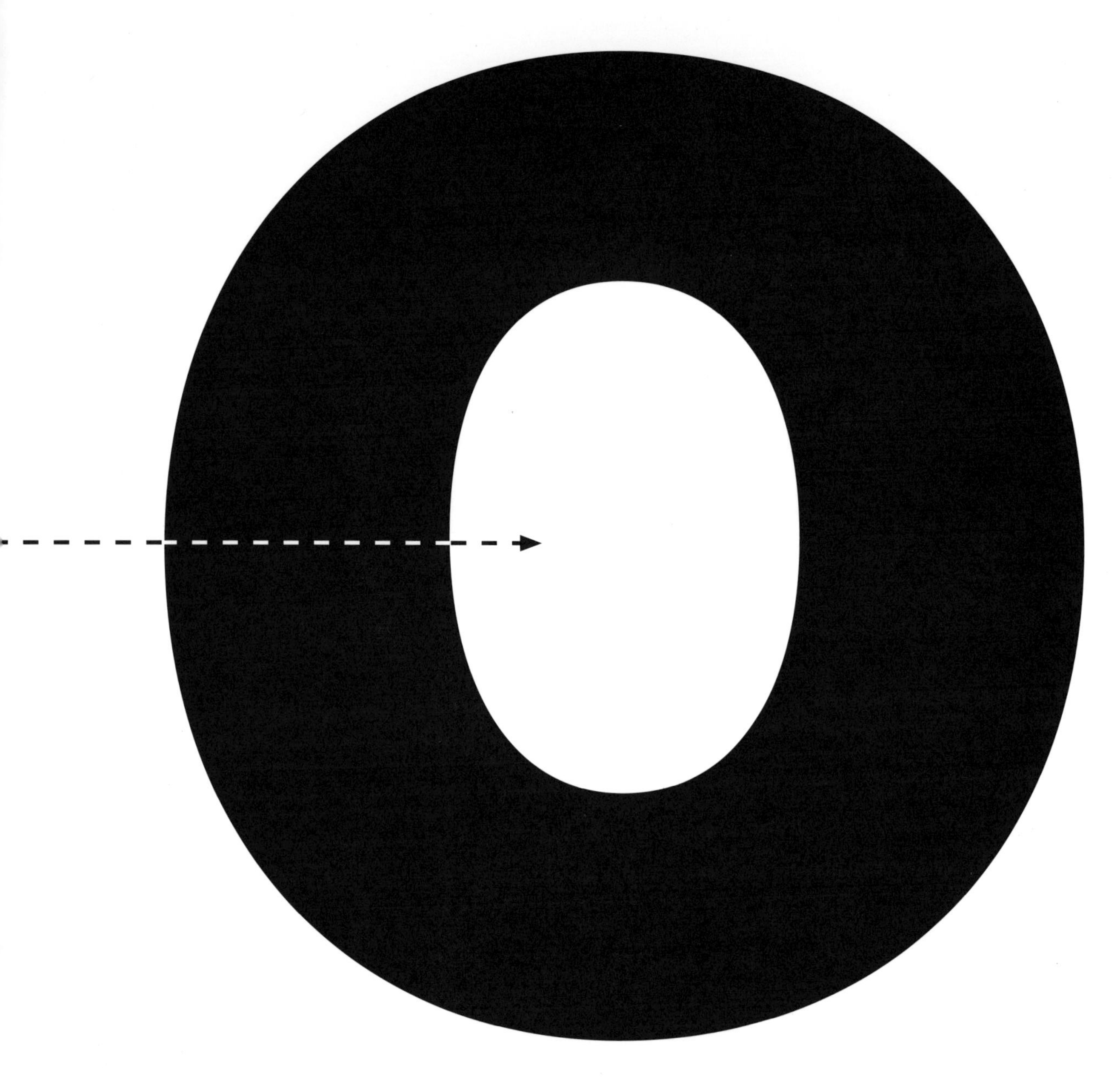

O is for **Obstacles**

It is okay to feel **O**verwhelmed
and **O**verburdened.

Other's **O**pinions are **O**ptional.
Orchestrate your **O**wn **O**asis.

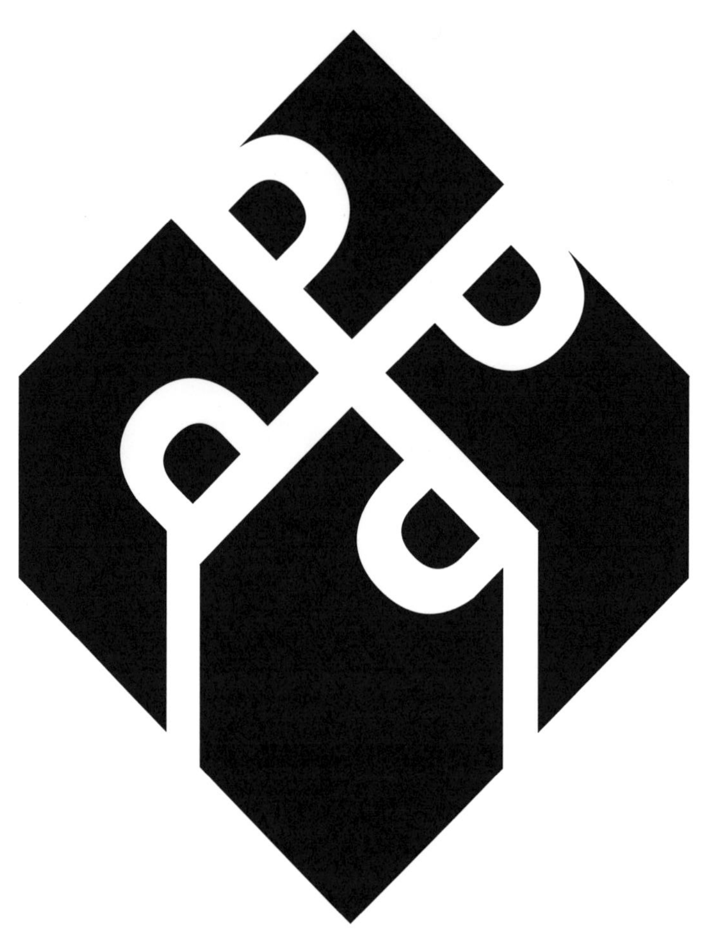

P is for **Packages of mindfulness**

It is okay to feel **P**erplexed and **P**uzzled.

Pen a note to yourself from your loved one.
Pent-up emotions block **P**ersonal development.

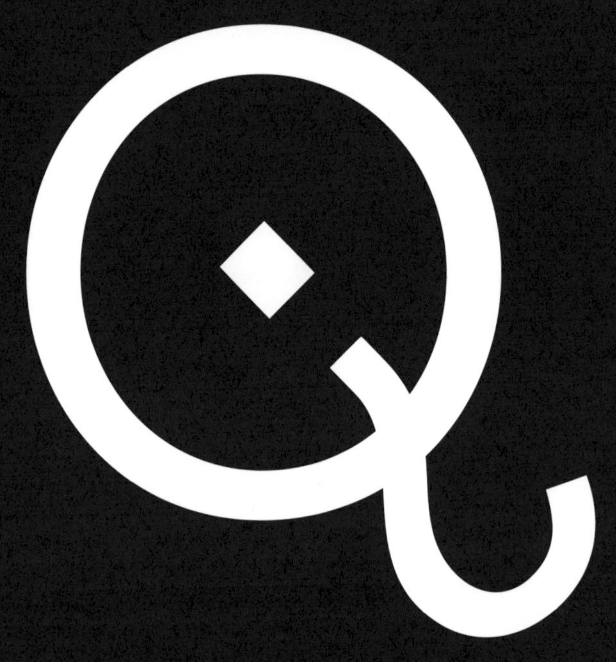

Q is for **Qualm**

It is okay to **Q**uestion.

Qwest into your spirituality.
Quiet lulls calm.

Я

R is for **Remembering**

It is okay to feel **R**eminiscent as memories live-on.

Rearview mirrors offer solace to griefviews. **R**each into yesterday, which is part of today, and a portion of tomorrow.

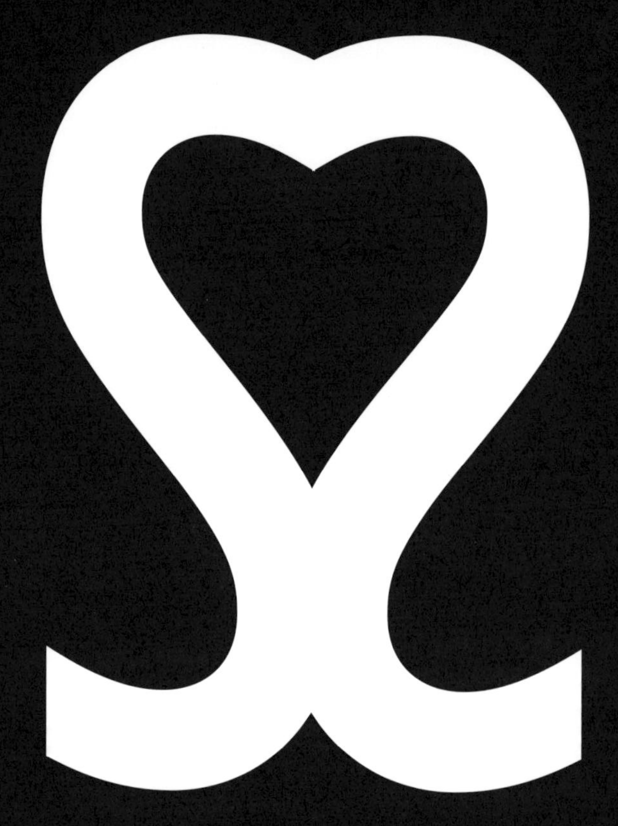

S is for **Safekeeping**

It is okay to feel **S**cared your loved one
may be forgotten.

Storytell your loss.
Soak up your **S**orrow so it can **S**often.

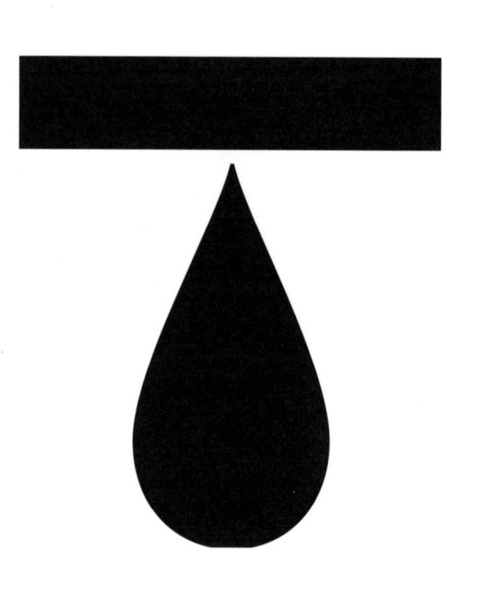

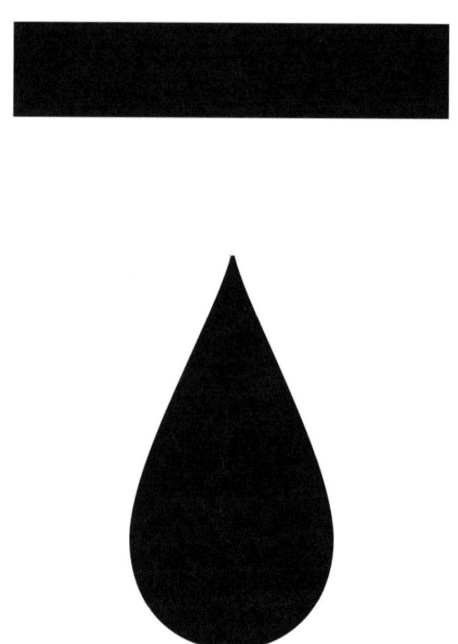

T is for **Tears**

It is okay to cry **T**oday and **T**omorrow.

Touch their picture.
Tears are waterfalls from the heart.

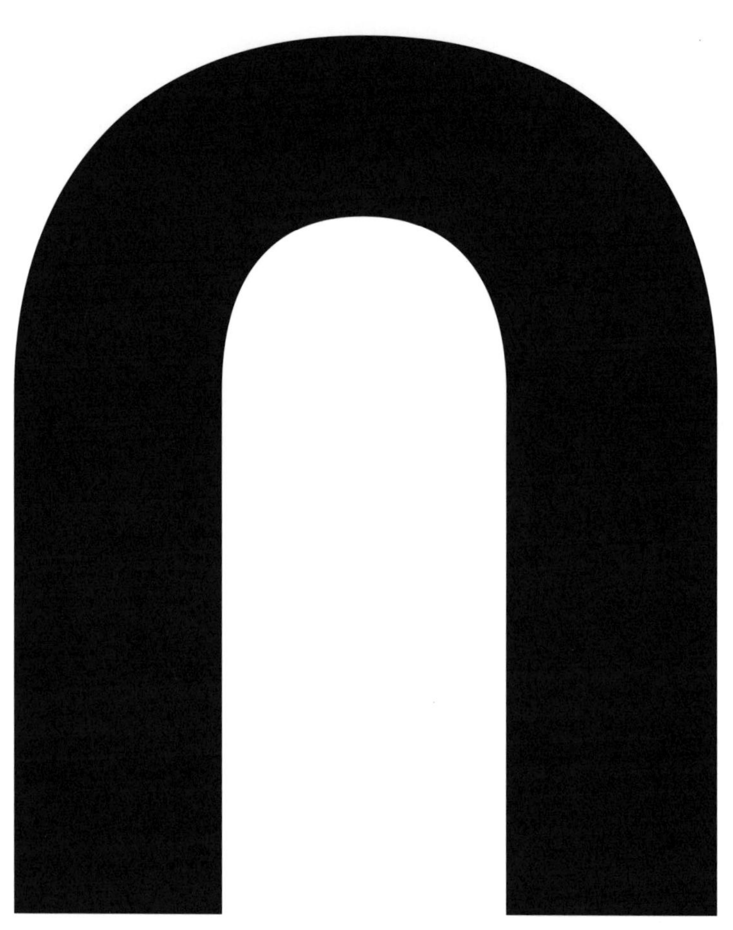

U is for **Upheaval**

It is okay to feel **U**prooted
in an **U**nknown world.

Unwind a tape measure and measure
your scale of sadness.
Unlocking your grief acknowledges
its importance.

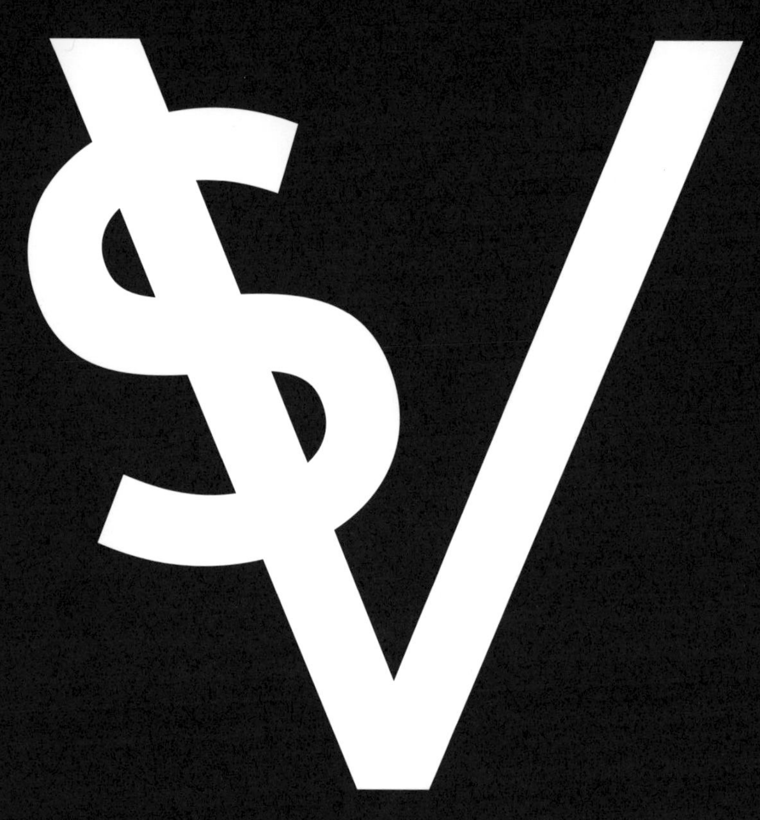

V is for **Valuable**

It is okay to feel **V**ulnerable.

Voice a compliment to yourself.
Visions of support from your heart are **V**ital.

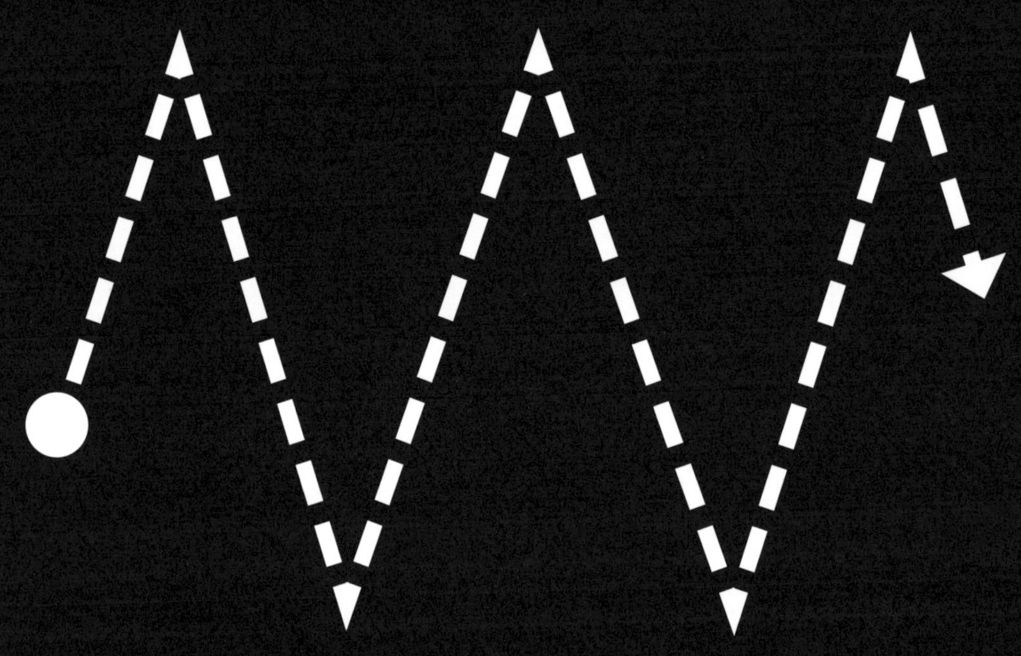

W is for **Wondering**

It is okay to feel **W**orried and **W**istful.

Wear a hat.
Warm your mind while climbing
the **W**all of Grief.

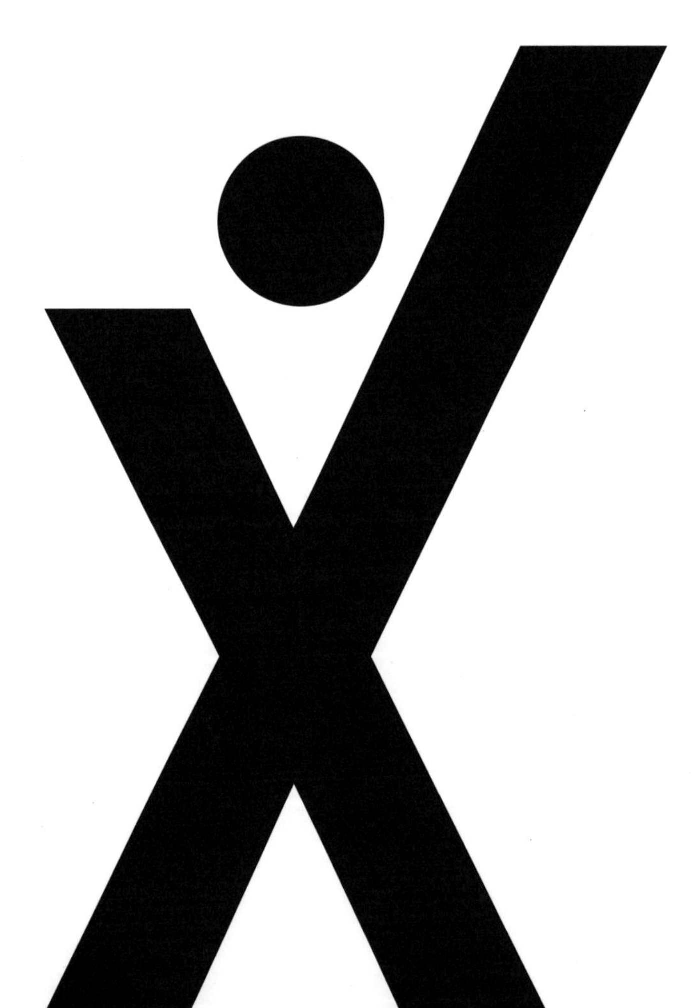

X is for **eXtraordinary**

It is okay to feel e**X**clusive.

e**X**periment with clay.
e**X**plore your hope rainbow.

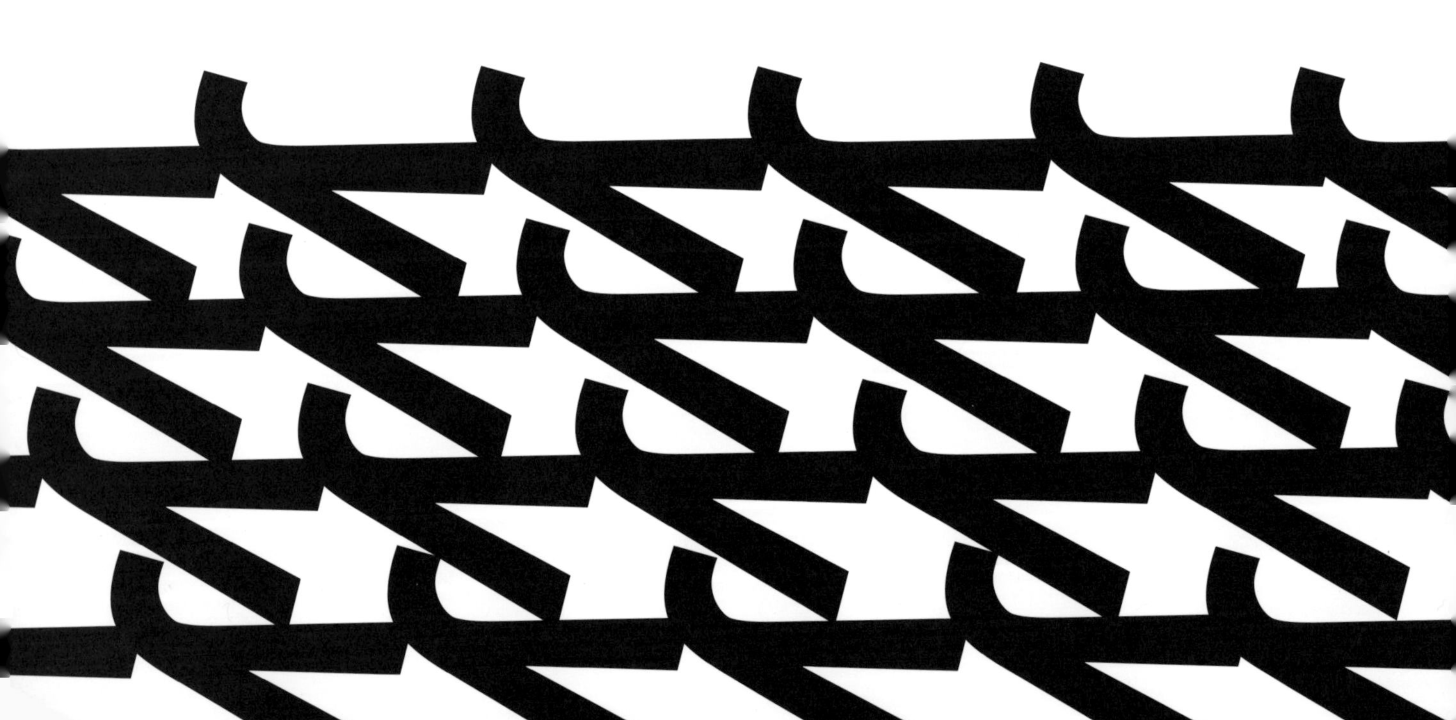

Y is for **Yearning**

It is okay to ride the
"Wish **Y**ou Were Here" **Y**acht.

Yelp like a coyote.
Yells communicate **Y**our agony.

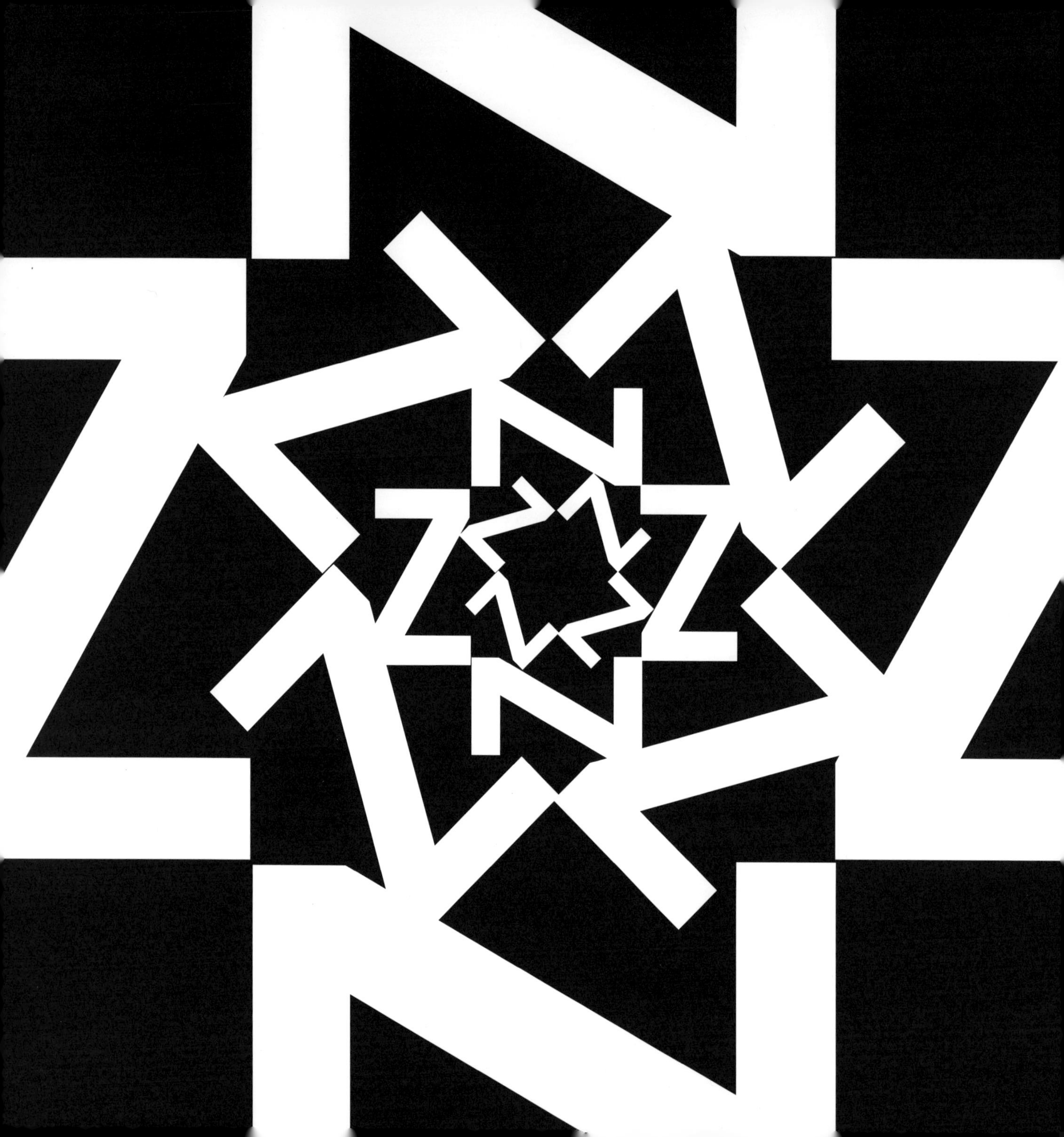

Z is for **Zones of grief**

It is okay to feel like a **Z**ombie.

Zoo visits are intriguing.
Zap your personal cages and re-discover **Z**eal.

Your life colors will someday reappear
in newly-mixed hues of forward-looking hope.

And what "once was" will be stored
in soul-nourishing corners of your heart.